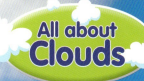

What Are CUMULUS CLOUDS?

Lynn Peppas

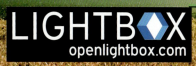

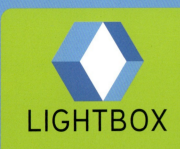

LIGHTBOX

Go to
www.openlightbox.com
and enter this book's
unique code.

ACCESS CODE

LBXX8337

Lightbox is an all-inclusive digital solution for the teaching and learning of curriculum topics in an original, groundbreaking way. Lightbox is based on National Curriculum Standards.

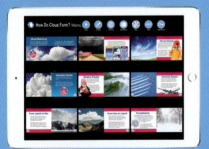

OPTIMIZED FOR
✓ TABLETS
✓ WHITEBOARDS
✓ COMPUTERS
✓ AND MUCH MORE!

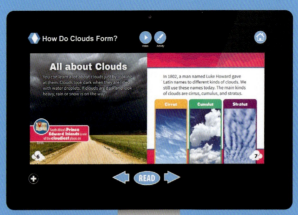

Copyright © 2021 Smartbook Media Inc. All rights reserved.

STANDARD FEATURES OF LIGHTBOX

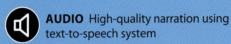
AUDIO High-quality narration using text-to-speech system

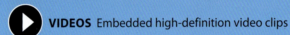
VIDEOS Embedded high-definition video clips

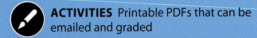
ACTIVITIES Printable PDFs that can be emailed and graded

WEBLINKS Curated links to external, child-safe resources

SLIDESHOWS Pictorial overviews of key concepts

INTERACTIVE MAPS Interactive maps and aerial satellite imagery

QUIZZES Ten multiple choice questions that are automatically graded and emailed for teacher assessment

KEY WORDS Matching key concepts to their definitions

VIDEOS
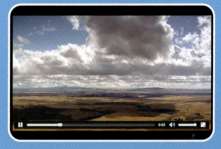

WEBLINKS
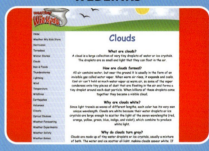

SLIDESHOWS
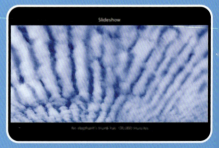

QUIZZES
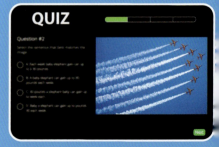

What Are CUMULUS CLOUDS?

Contents

- 2   Lightbox Access Code
- 4   Watching Clouds
- 6   All about Clouds
- 8   Cloud Heights
- 10 What Are Cumulus Clouds?
- 12 Cumulus Heights
- 14 Cumulus Weather
- 16 Moved by the Wind
- 18 The Water Cycle
- 20 Precipitation
- 22 Quiz
- 24 Key Words

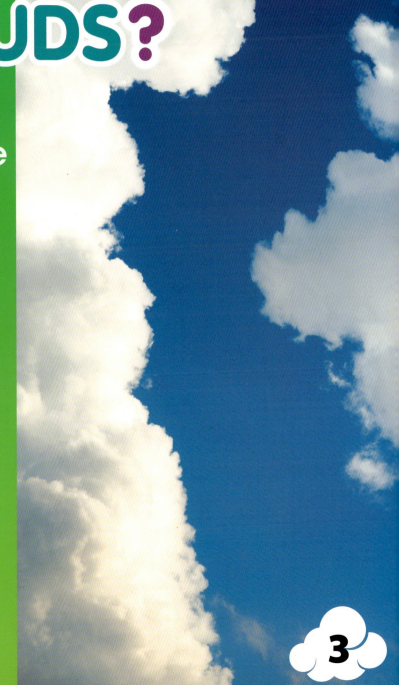

Watching Clouds

Watching clouds in the sky is like watching a magic show. Clouds **constantly change shape**. Some even disappear right before your eyes.

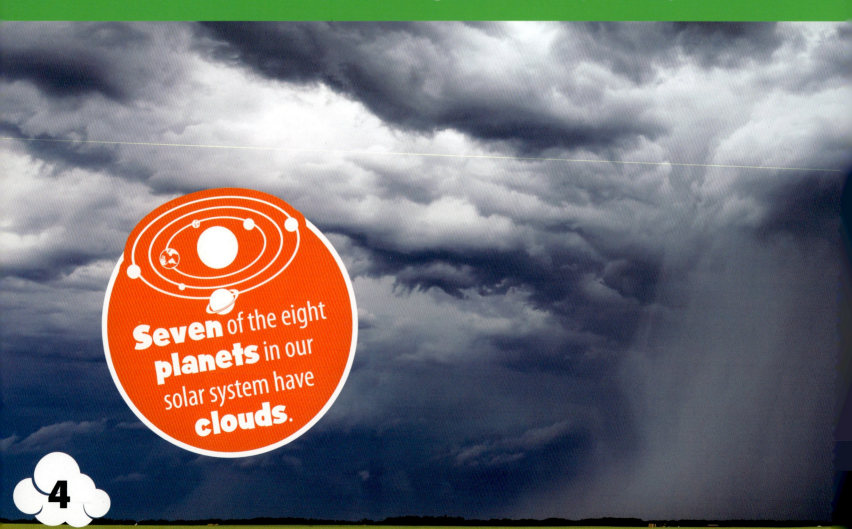

Seven of the eight **planets** in our solar system have **clouds**.

Clouds give clues as to what the **weather** will be like. Different kinds of clouds bring **different kinds of weather**.

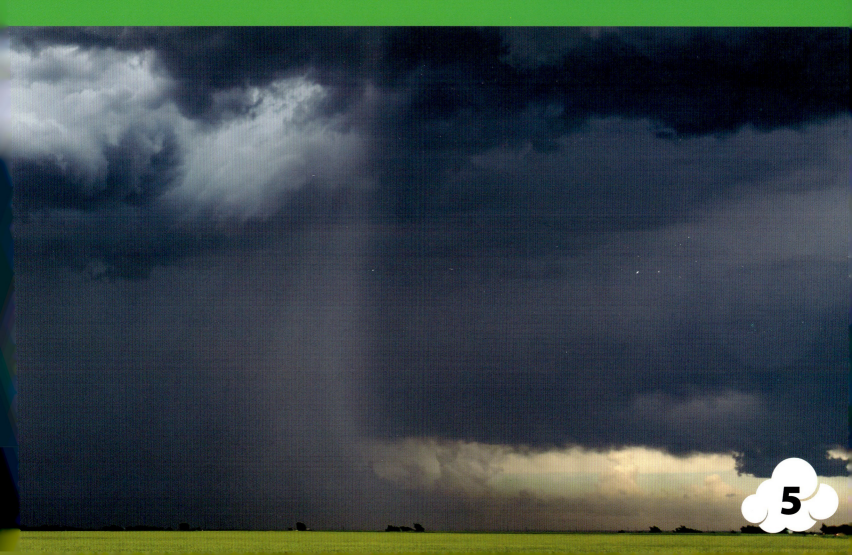

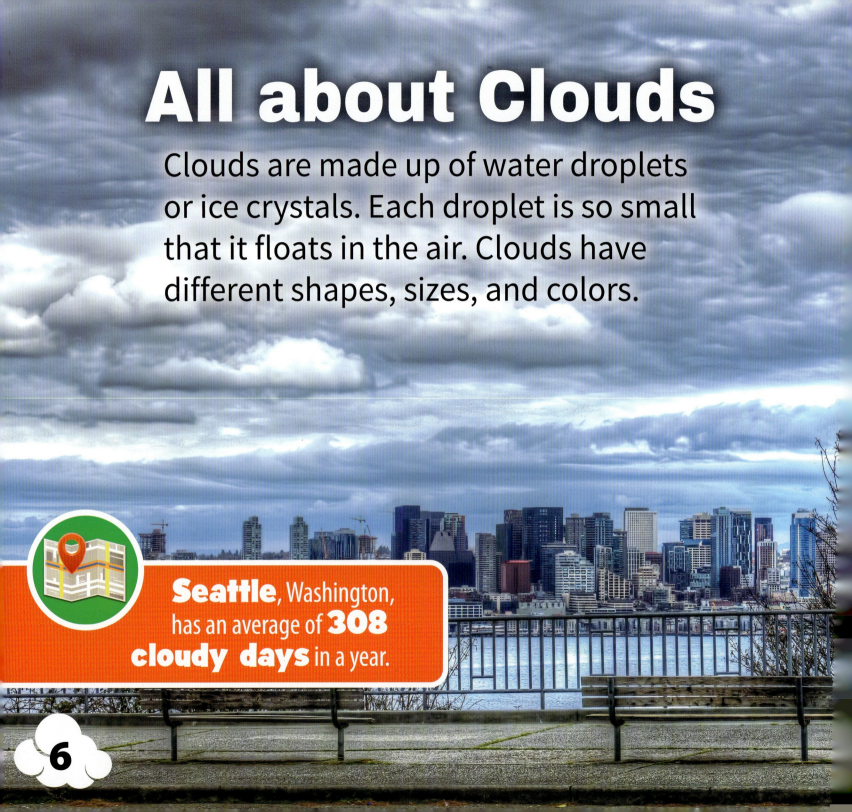

All about Clouds

Clouds are made up of water droplets or ice crystals. Each droplet is so small that it floats in the air. Clouds have different shapes, sizes, and colors.

Seattle, Washington, has an average of **308 cloudy days** in a year.

More than 200 years ago, a man called Luke Howard named different clouds by their shapes. The three main kinds of clouds are cirrus, cumulus, and stratus clouds.

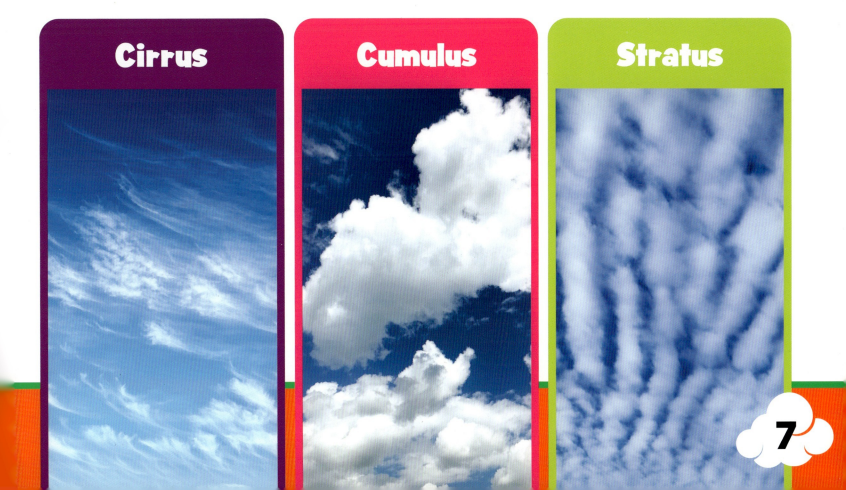

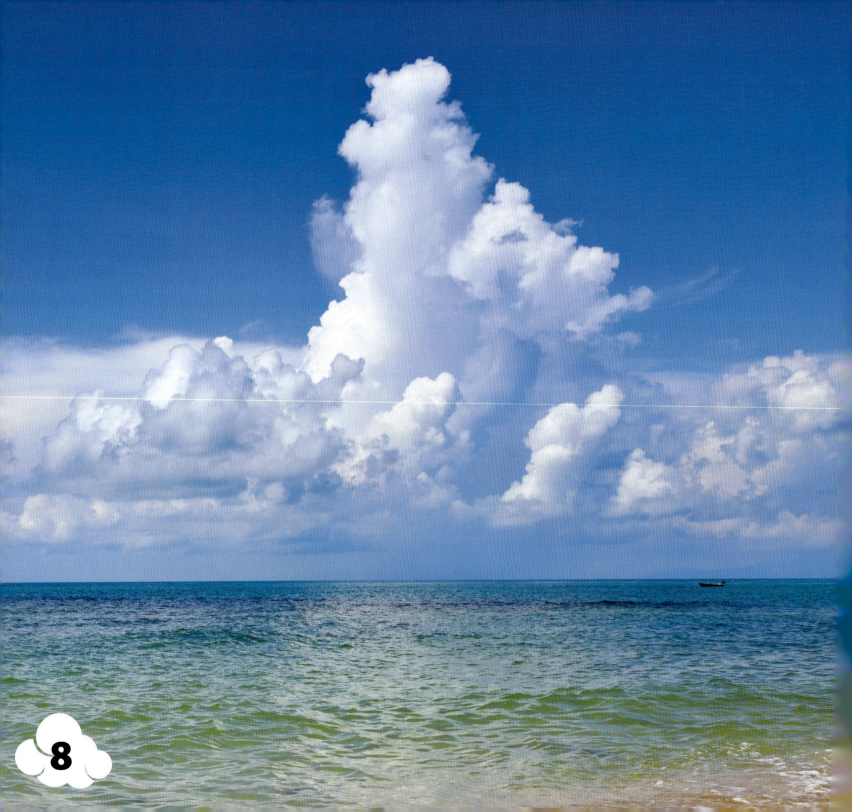

Cloud Heights

Some clouds form high in the sky. The highest clouds have names that start with "cirro."

Other kinds of clouds form so low that they touch the ground. Low clouds have "strato" in their names. Clouds that form in the middle of the sky have names that begin with "alto."

What Are Cumulus Clouds?

Cumulus clouds are bright white clouds with puffy tops and flat bottoms. These clouds look like floating piles of cotton balls. They are made up of tiny water droplets.

Most cumulus clouds form about 1 mile above Earth's surface. At this height, the air is usually warm enough to let the cloud gather more droplets and grow larger.

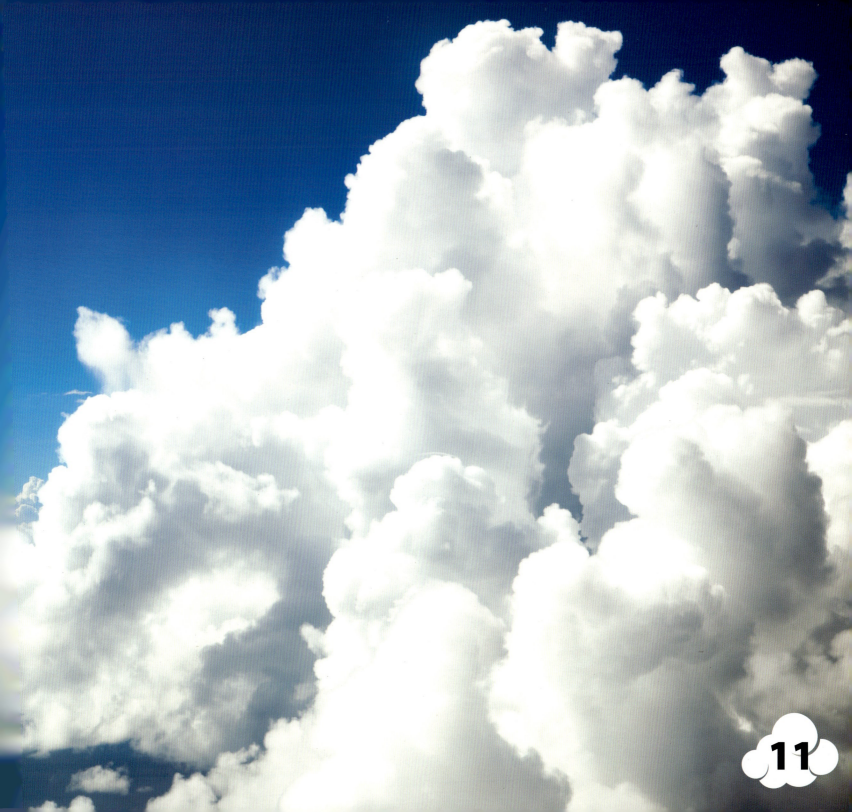

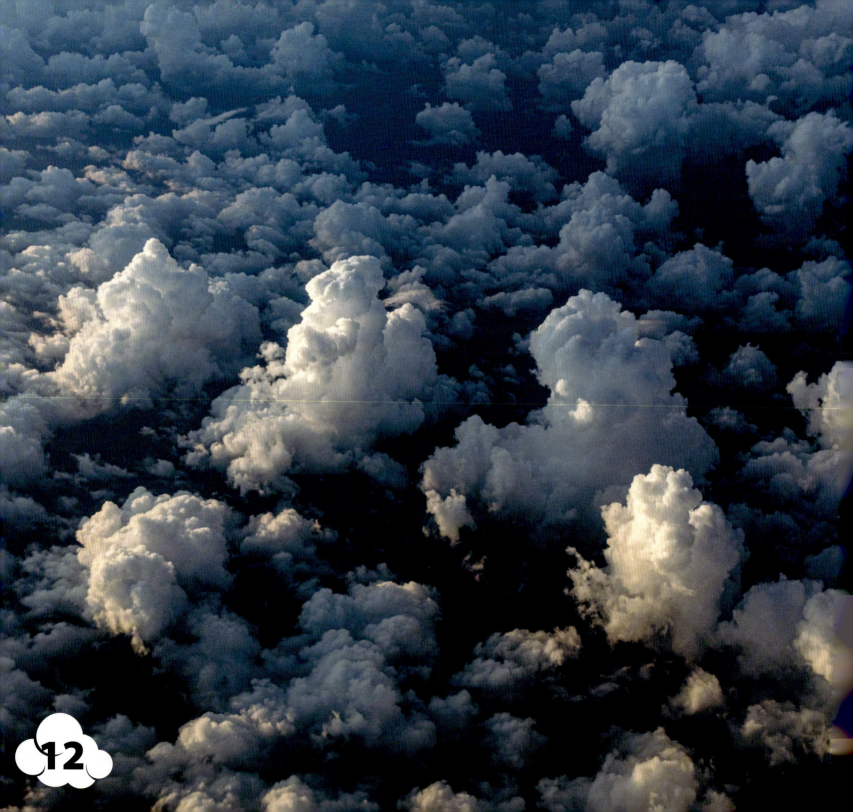

Cumulus Heights

Cumulus clouds that form low in the sky are called stratocumulus clouds. Stratocumulus clouds are lumpy and gray. Altocumulus clouds are cumulus clouds that form in the middle of the sky.

Cirrocumulus clouds are the highest-forming cumulus clouds in the sky. The air at this height is very cold. Because of this, cirrocumulus clouds are made up of ice crystals.

Cumulus Weather

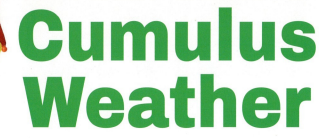

Cumulus clouds are sometimes called "fair-weather clouds." When you see them, the weather is usually bright and pleasant.

If you see cumulus clouds growing taller and darker, beware! The cumulus cloud may be changing into a cumulonimbus cloud. This is a sign that a storm is on its way.

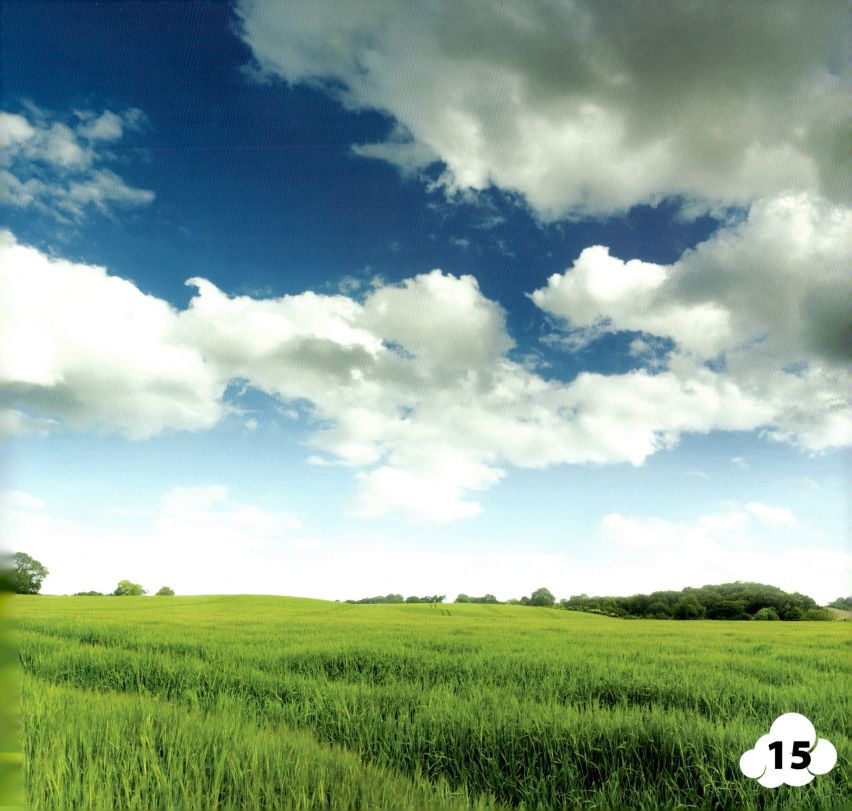

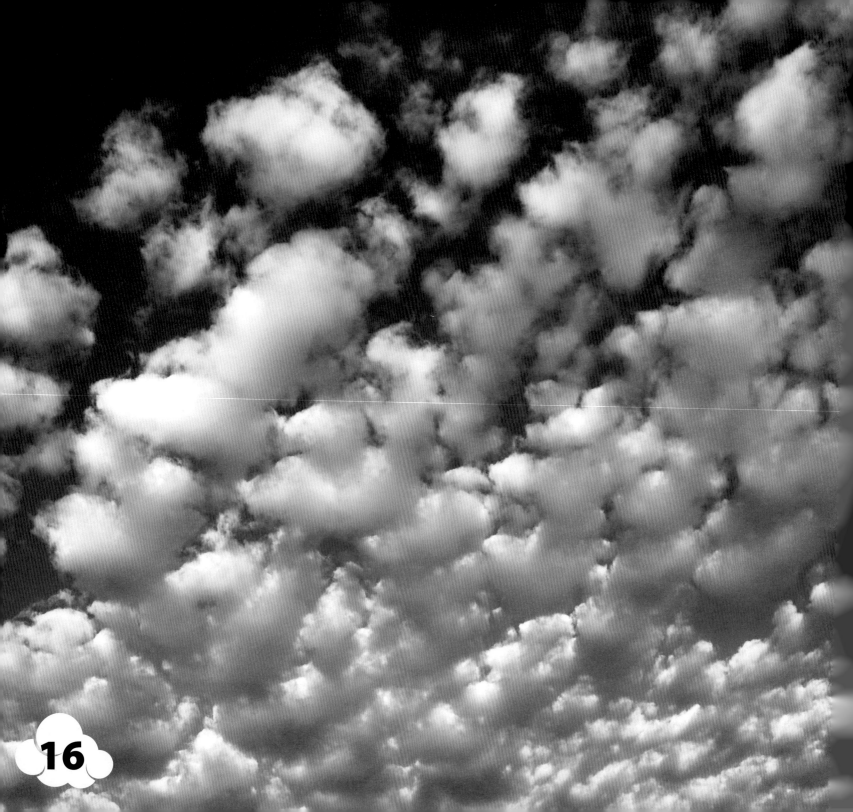

Moved by the Wind

Cumulus clouds move and change. Like all clouds, they are moved by wind. Wind is moving air. Sometimes, strong winds push cumulus clouds higher in the sky, turning them into altocumulus clouds.

Altocumulus clouds are usually light gray. They can be a sign that rainy weather is on its way.

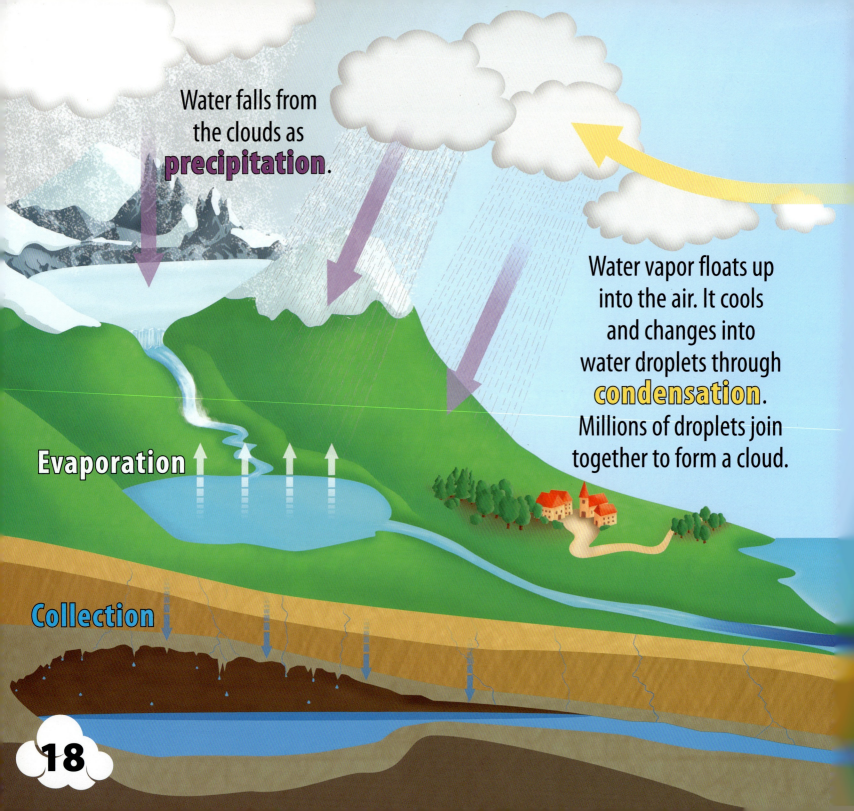

The Water Cycle

The water cycle describes how water moves around Earth. Clouds are an important part of this cycle.

The Sun heats the water in oceans, lakes, and rivers. Heat makes some of the water **evaporate**, or change into water vapor.

Collection

Precipitation

Precipitation is rain, snow, or other forms of water that fall from clouds. Cumulonimbus clouds produce heavy precipitation.

These clouds are dark and dense, bringing rain, thunder, and lightning. They are also the only clouds that make hail. All thunderstorms come from cumulonimbus clouds.

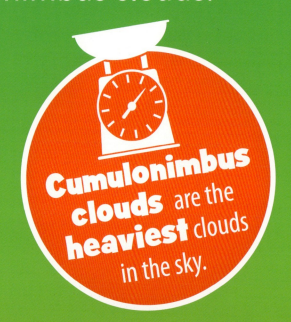

Cumulonimbus clouds are the heaviest clouds in the sky.

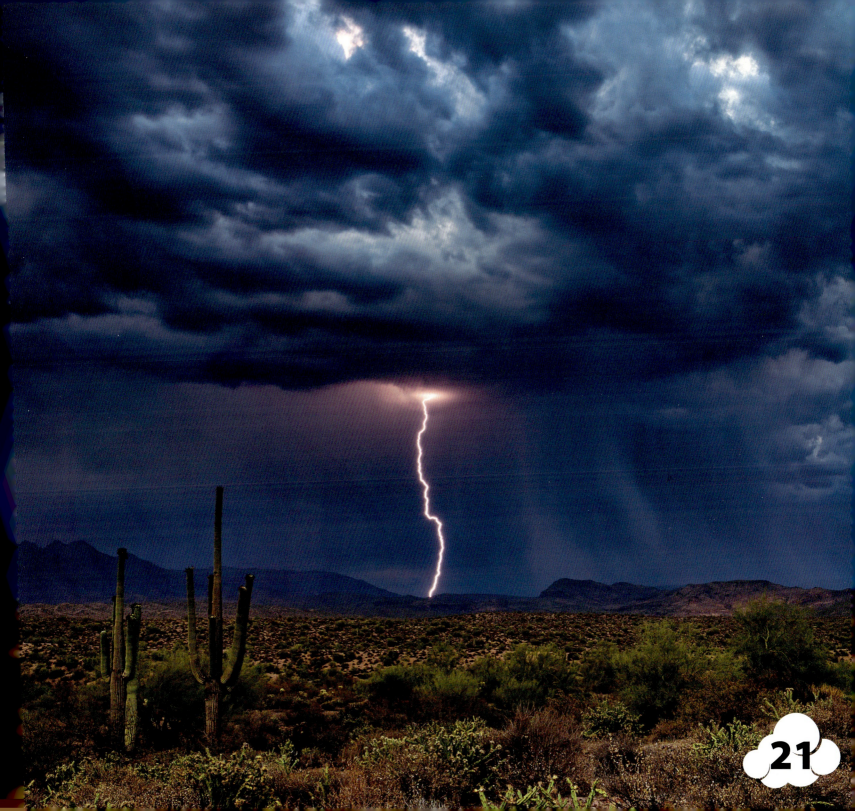

Quiz

Can you name the types of clouds in these pictures?

A. Cirrus
B. Cumulus
C. Stratus
D. Altocumulus
E. Cumulonimbus

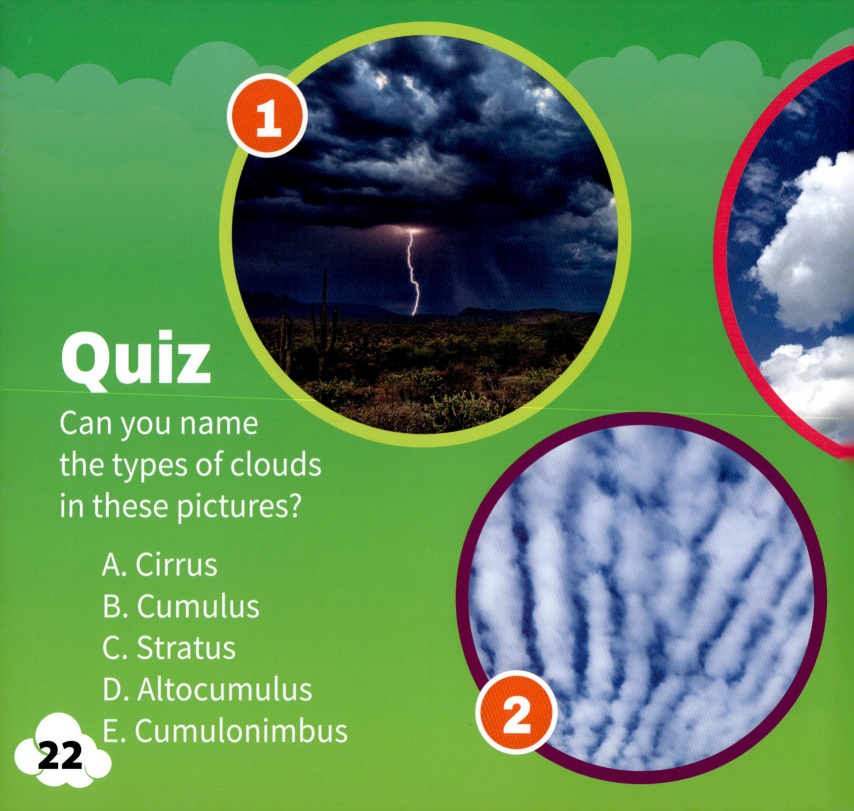

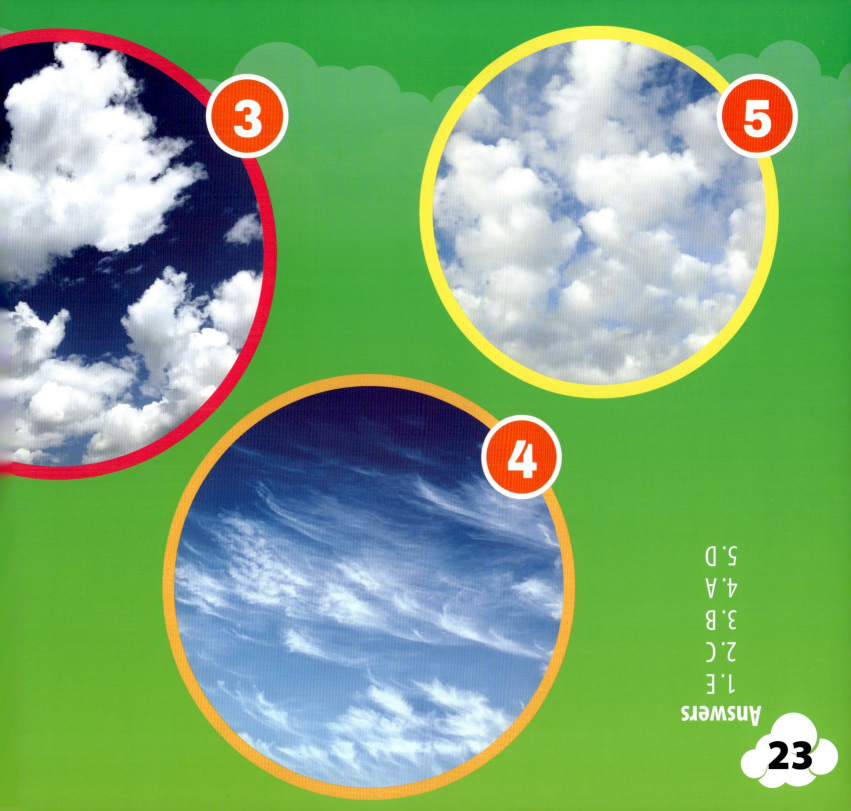

Answers
1. E
2. C
3. B
4. A
5. D

23

KEY WORDS

Research has shown that as much as 65 percent of all written material published in English is made up of 300 words. These 300 words cannot be taught using pictures or learned by sounding them out. They must be recognized by sight. This book contains 95 common sight words to help young readers improve their reading fluency and comprehension. This book also teaches young readers several important content words, such as proper nouns. These words are paired with pictures to aid in learning and improve understanding.

Page	Sight Words First Appearance
4	a, before, change, even, eyes, have, in, is, like, of, our, right, show, some, the, your
5	as, be, different, give, kinds, to, what, will
6	about, air, all, an, and, are, days, each, has, it, made, or, small, so, that, up, water, year
7	by, man, more, than, their, three
9	begin, high, names, other, start, they, with
10	above, at, Earth, enough, grow, let, look, mile, most, these, this, through, white
13	because, very
14	if, into, its, on, see, sometimes, them, way, when, you
17	can, light, move
18	from, through, together
19	around, how, important, makes, part, rivers
20	also, come, only

Page	Content Words First Appearance
4	clouds, planets, shape, sky, solar system
5	clues, weather
6	average, colors, ice crystals, Seattle, sizes, Washington, droplets
7	cirrus, cumulus, Luke Howard, stratus
9	"alto," "cirro," ground, heights, "strato"
10	cotton balls, flat bottoms, puffy tops, surface, piles, water cycle
13	altocumulus, cirrocumulus, stratocumulus
14	cumulonimbus, "fair-weather clouds," sign, storm
17	wind
18	collection, condensation, evaporation, precipitation, water vapor
19	heat, lakes, oceans, Sun
20	hail, lightning, rain, snow, thunder, thunderstorms

Published by Smartbook Media Inc.
350 5th Avenue, 59th Floor New York, NY 10118
Website: www.openlightbox.com

Copyright ©2021 Smartbook Media Inc.
All rights reserved. No part of this publication may be reproduced, stored in a retrieval system, or transmitted in any form or by any means, electronic, mechanical, photocopying, recording, or otherwise, without the prior written permission of the publisher.

Library of Congress Control Number: 2020936913

ISBN 978-1-5105-5556-3 (hardcover)
ISBN 978-1-5105-5557-0 (multi-user eBook)

Printed in Guangzhou, China
1 2 3 4 5 6 7 8 9 0   24 23 22 21 20

042020
110819

Project Coordinator: Priyanka Das
Designer: Ana María Vidal

Every reasonable effort has been made to trace ownership and to obtain permission to reprint copyright material. The publisher would be pleased to have any errors or omissions brought to its attention so that they may be corrected in subsequent printings.

The publisher acknowledges Alamy, Getty Images, and iStock as the primary image suppliers for this title.

First published by Crabtree Publishing Company in 2012.